"Destruction From Within"

= = =

Trump's Wall
vs
America's Drugs-Epidemic

= = =

"Drugs now kill more people in America than cars and guns!"

William James Moore

The Serenity Prayer"

*"**God** grant me the . . .*
*****Serenity** to accept the things I cannot change;*
*****Courage** to change the things I can; and*
*****Wisdom** to know the difference."*

– Reinhold Niebuhr (1892–1971)

= = =

Dedication

To the Countless Struggling with Addictions;
Their Families; and Affected Others

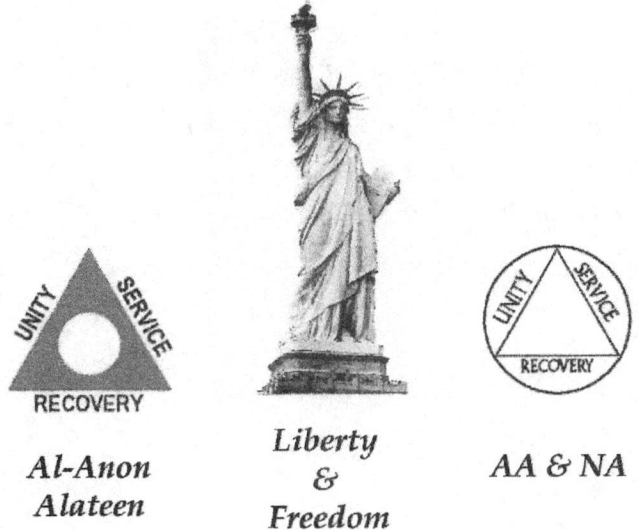

Al-Anon
Alateen

Liberty
&
Freedom

AA & NA

"In the beginning God created the heaven and the earth."
— Genesis 1:1

THE CROSS ROOM

The young man was at the end of his rope.
Seeing no way out, he dropped to his knees in prayer.
"Lord, I can't go on," he said.
"I have too heavy a cross to bear."
The Lord replied,
"My son, if you can't bear its weight,
just place your cross inside this room.
Then open another door and pick any cross you wish."
The man was filled with relief.
"Thank you, Lord,"
he sighed, and did as he was told.
As he looked around the room he saw many different crosses;
some so large the tops were not visible.
Then he spotted a tiny cross leaning against a far wall.
"I'd like that one, Lord,"
he whispered. And the Lord replied,
"My son, that's the cross you brought in."

— Author Unknown

[The above, courtesy of "Greg & Osa"]

= = =

[Special Remarks: Obviously, the above story's special message applies to all of us—to all humankind world-wide. When life's problems seem overwhelming, if we would only look around and see what others are coping with, we may then consider ourselves far more fortunate than we imagined.]

Contents

Special Appreciation

≈

With My Love Always—

To "Ann, Jamie, Ryan, and Matthew"
From "James, Dad, & Papa"

= = =

Acknowledgements

The information shared herein was drawn from my and others' life experiences, observations, and research. Others to whom I am deeply appreciative for the shared enlightenment and access to crucially worthwhile information.

Preface

The universal struggles to experience love, joy, happiness, belonging, social relevance, longevity, freedom or relief from pain, etc., and various escapes from some of life's discomforting and sometimes harsh realities, have likely been with us since the beginning of humankind. Struggles also concerning the special challenges associated with self-perceived "uniqueness," suffered at times by many, if not all, of us in some manner.

And among the many responses to such age-old struggles has come an ever-growing arsenal of natural and man-made "substances." Some offering solutions and promise on one hand, while also harboring the many sufferings involved with addiction. For example, substances commonly called "drugs," "alcohol," "tobacco," "marijuana," "narcotics," and seemingly less stigmatizing and less threatening terms, such as "prescription medications," etc.

Substances used legally and illegally for a growing number or purposes, including but not limited to; recreation; relief of pain, ranging from the imagined to the most severe; stress relief or avoidance; treatment of diseases ranging from the common cold to the most painful and debilitating; capital punishment; performance enhancement; sedation; stimulation; and behavior control (such as, wrongfully and destructively preventing young children from behaving like "young children").

"Addictive substances" that (regardless of technical definition) are all nonetheless very much "mood and behavior altering." [*Think not? Then step into the shoes of anyone now abusing or attempting to withdraw from any addictive substance – yes, even alcohol, marijuana, tobacco, etc. Or, into the shoes of the family or other lives that drug-abuse impacts.*] Therefore, throughout this book, each and all such substances will simply and fittingly be referred to as **"addictive-drugs."** Whose use and abuse by millions can, and increasingly does, involve a thin line between a positive outcome and one of dependency, addiction, and death.

The types natural and man-made "addictive-drugs" are many and involve a long and complex history of world-wide scope. One entailing a depth of detail purposely not addressed herein. Nor is such detail required in order to grasp the truly devastating reality of America's "present and rapidly spreading" addictive-drugs epidemic. One fueled in large measure by both our natural and unrealistic cravings; a profit-driven drug industry; drug cartels; ignorance; apathy, complacency, denial, greed, fear; technology; and even well-intentioned physicians. A "self-destruction from within" that "Trump's Wall" and our nation's borders, regardless of how strong, will not alone shield us from. An ever-spreading epidemic of tragedy from which no individual, family, group, age, race, religion, sexual orientation, political affiliation, or other population demographic is immune!

= = =

"There is no chemical solution to a spiritual problem."

– anonymous

Introduction

> *"America will never be destroyed from the outside. If we falter and lose our freedoms, it will be because we destroyed ourselves.* —Abraham Lincoln (1809–1865), 16th U.S. President

Dear Reader,

The United States first outlawed "addictive-drugs" in the early 1900s. The Food and Drugs Act of 1906 was the beginning of over 200 laws regarding public health and consumer protections. Over 100 years later, our nation is struggling with an ever-growing, out-of-control, "addictive-drugs epidemic"!

Persons reasonably attuned to current events have at least heard about the "illegal flow" of drugs, cash, guns, people, etc., into our country. Especially through our southern border. And persons in touch with any sense of reality also have some basic appreciation of the serious threats posed by trafficking. Of common awareness also is President Trump's campaign pledge to "build a wall" on our southern border, as a major defensive measure against drug-trafficking, illegal immigration, and other border-related threats.

This writer is among our nation's millions of strong supporters of "Trump's wall" and of other effective measures to secure and control our nation's borders. For secured-borders, along with a common-language (English in the U.S.), and common-culture (Judeo Christian in the U.S.), are among the critical foundation blocks for any nation's long survival.

However, secured borders will not alone protect us from **"destruction from within"**! From self-destructive behaviors such as, but not limited to, our craving for, dependency upon, and addiction to: drugs of all types; cheap labor for big and small businesses; cheap products for the insatiable American consumer; people with unsatisfied "wants and needs" to justify the services and agendas of various government programs and charitable institutions; and people who can be swayed to forever join the ranks of robot-voters for a particular political party; etc.

It is not only noteworthy, but should also serve as a wake-up call, that the Mexican drug-cartels are not flooding our country with "wheels for covered wagons of years long past." For, it is "addictive-drugs" that we crave, have dependency upon, and addiction to—and not "wheels for covered wagons"!

Nor, are our U.S. shopping malls filled with protestors demanding "made in the U.S.A." products, as we freely spend our money on merchandise made by underpaid (often under-aged and enslaved) foreign workers, as we at the same time rant about lost jobs in America.

And in contrast to the countless striving for legal and illegal entry into the into the U.S., none are likewise lined up outside the borders of North Korea, Iran, Syria, etc. For, within the borders of such dictator nations, there is no government-tolerated demand or tolerance for people in search of liberty, freedom, opportunity, or charity. Or for offended or otherwise misguided souls seeking a personal "safe space" or other special considerations at the expense of others.

However, returning to "Trump's wall" — no **"clear-headed thinking"** would ever seriously question that effectively secured borders are needed for survival against threats from the **"outside."** Nor would any "clear-headed thinking" doubt the need for good judgement and personal responsibility in dealing with threats posed from **"within."** None the least the threat posed by our nation's rapidly spreading "addictive-drugs epidemic." Fueled not by an external enemy alone, but ultimately by demands from "within." From within our borders — and ourselves! Fueled by cravings for freedom from physical and mental pain; cravings to experience unnatural joy and euphoria; cravings to escape some of the unpleasant, and at times overwhelming, realities of life.

However, the same "clear-headed thinking" needed to successfully deal with our nation's addictive-drugs epidemic, is threatened by the very nature of epidemic itself. By the ability of "addictive-drugs" to negatively interfere with our judgement and decision making. Leaving millions caught in the jaws of drug abuse, dependency, and addiction, with their mental capacity (good judgement) needed to escape severely challenged. Leaving them, their families, and affected others, with a progressively worsening suffering. From which no individual, family, group, occupation, position of power or influence, age, race, religion, sexual orientation, political affiliation, or other population demographic, has immunity!

It is a most sincere wish and aim that book provide meaningful support to the many ongoing battles against our nation's addictive-drugs epidemic. A deep desire in clear awareness of a most clear reality — that this relatively limited writing is but a speck of sand on a vast beach of other available works. Other information of much more depth and detail, expressed in a growing number of books, websites, and other sources. A readily available vast treasure of enlightening material and points of contact for an array of drug-abuse support services.

In our respective gift-of-life journeys and support against our country's many threats, may we be blessed with **sound judgement and responsible conduct**. Fueled by the **wisdom** and **willingness** to do the right thing on behalf of the greater good. On behalf of our nation, critically burdened by what has now truly become an "addictive-drugs epidemic" — many years in the making.

— William James Moore

= = =

"We cannot solve our problems with the same thinking we used when we created them." — Albert Einstein (1879-1955)

America's "Drugs-Epidemic": How Bad Is It?

Since 2002, over 500,000 people in the U.S. have died from drug over-doses. That's a half-million people – over an average of 35,000 per year – at least 1 drug-overdose death every 15 minutes!

It is a rapidly growing reality that someone in your family has been or will be touched by the devastation of drug abuse, dependency, and addiction. And/or that your family knows of someone who has – or will be!

This Section includes various random-listed statistics, news headlines, and other information regarding our nation's drug-epidemic. While only a very limited glimpse at the growing magnitude that exists, any serious review of the following should provide the reader with a meaningful grasp of the truly serious extent of our country's drug-epidemic. If not, it is unlikely that additional written words would be helpful towards such end, regardless of content, format, or source.

= = =

Drug overdose is now the **"leading cause"** of accidental death in the U.S. More Americans are now being killed by drugs than automobiles and guns!

In 2015 some 35,092 were killed in automobile accidents; about 12,942 people died from gun homicide, accidental shooting, or murder and suicide. During same year, at least **55,403** died from lethal drug overdoses.

Although involving an array of drugs, "opioids" are leading our nation's drug-epidemic. With, during the above same YR 2015 time frame, at least 20,101 overdose deaths from prescription pain relievers, and more than 12,990 overdose deaths from heroin.

Since 1999, every racial demographic has suffered an increase in drug overdoses. Since 2010, the drug overdose death rate of African-Americans has increased over 200 percent; the Latino death rate by almost 140 percent. With drug overdose death rates of Whites and Native Americans more than doubling that of African-Americans and Latinos by 2014.

From 1999 to 2014 heroin-related deaths increased 439 percent, having tripled in five years and quintupled in ten years. America's heroin and opioid epidemic death rates now compare to those suffered from AIDS in the 1990s.

Doctors wrote at about 76 million opioid prescriptions in 1991 (for hydrocodone and oxycodone products, etc.). A number that by 2011 had almost tripled to 219 million. A dramatic increase made critically more threatening by drug cartels flooding the U.S. with heroin. Providing a cheaper, more potent, and in many cases easier to obtain source than prescription pain medications. In the four years of 2005–2009, Mexican heroin production increased more than six-times to an estimated 8 metric tons.

Opioid prescriptions vary considerably by state. During the 2012 timeframe, doctors in Hawaii wrote 52 opioid prescriptions per every 100 people; whereas Alabama doctors wrote 143 per 100 people. And as shown by the following Table, in 2012 twelve states had more opioid prescriptions than people!

Twelve States With More Opioid Pain-reliever Prescriptions Than People in 2012		
State/Opioid Prescriptions (Per 100 People)		**State/Opioid Prescriptions (Per 100 People)**
Alabama: 142.9		Louisiana: 118
Tennessee: 142.8		Arkansas: 115.8
West Virginia: 137.6		Indiana: 109.1
Kentucky: 128.4		Michigan: 107
Oklahoma: 127.8		South Carolina: 101.8
Mississippi: 120.3		Ohio: 100.1
Source: Centers of Disease Control & Prevention (CDC) - 2012 data		

Opioid prescriptions more than tripled nationwide between 1999 and 2014. In 2014, sixty-one percent of all U.S. drug overdose deaths involved opioids.

America's drug-abuse epidemic touches every age group.

Overdose Deaths by Age in 2014				
Age (Years)	**Deaths Per 100,000**			
	From Heroin		**From Opioids**	
15-24	3.3		3.1	
25-34	8		9	
35-44	**5.9**		10.3	
45-54	4.7		**11.7**	
55-64	2.7		8.5	
65-74	0.5		2.7	
Source: Centers for Disease Control & Prevention (CDC)				

Americans make up less than **5 percent** of the world's population but consume about **80 percent** of the world's prescription opioids. For example, the U.S. accounts for almost 100 percent of the world total for hydrocodone (e.g., Vicodin) and 81 percent for oxycodone (e.g., Percocet).

"The Cost"

Estimates of total overall **"yearly costs"** of substance abuse in the U.S. — including health-and-crime-related costs and lost productivity costs — exceed $600 billion. This includes about $193 billion from illicit (illegal) drugs; $193 billion from tobacco; and $235 billion from alcohol. And, as alarming as these statistics are (or should be), they do not fully take into consideration the "overall" devastating impact to public health and safety from drug abuse and addiction. For example, not included in, nor measurable by, these "dollar costs," is the destruction of families; loss of employment; failures in school; domestic violence; child abuse; and related pain, suffering, and lost hopes and dreams.

"Painkillers Are Not The Only Problem"

This and the following Section has purposely focused a lot on opioid prescription **painkillers** (such as, hydrocodone and oxycodone products) and the illegal drug heroin. Nevertheless, it is important to note that such are not the only drugs whose use has skyrocketed the past 15 years or so. For example, as reported by TIME in March of 2016, and using the same Center of Disease Control database that tracks the growth in fatal opioid and heroin overdoses, TIME collected data on cocaine, benzodiazepines (**sedatives** like Valium and Xanax) and **stimulants** like crystal meth. TIME's research found that all three categories (**painkillers, sedatives, and stimulants**) have risen dramatically since the year 2000.

However, in terms of abuse and mortality, "opioids" account for the greatest part of our nation's prescription-drug abuse problem. In the early part of the 21st century deaths related to prescription opioids began rising. And, by around 2002, death certificates began listing "opioid analgesic poisoning" as the cause of death more often than heroin or cocaine. While addictive-drug use is highest among people in their late teens and twenties, drug use is increasing among people in their fifties and early sixties. An increase in part due to aging of baby-boomers, whose illegal drug use have been historically higher than that of previous generations. In the first half of the 20th century it took around 50 years for the rate of heart disease to double in the U.S.; it has taken drug-related deaths but a fraction of that time!

And, if we have not yet grasped the truly serious nature of our nation's **addictive-drugs epidemic**, the following shameful tragedy, taken in part from a CNN reporting, dated September 16, 2016, should help enlighten us:

Re: *"In America's drug death capital: How heroin is scarring the next generation:* Huntington, West Virginia (CNN): Sara Murray tends to two dozen babies in the neonatal therapeutic unit at Cabell Huntington Hospital. They shake. They vomit. Their inconsolable, high-pitched screams pierce the air. The symptoms can last for hours, days or months. Graceful and soft-spoken, Murray is a seasoned nurse tirelessly defending the innocent. But even she gets worn down. On difficult days, she seeks a moment of refuge behind her desk and wonders: How did we get here? These babies -- her babies -- are the youngest, most vulnerable victims of a raging epidemic. They are heroin babies, **born addicted**. Her third-floor unit, a calm and quiet space with dim lighting, is meant to accommodate 12 babies, but it's been two years since the numbers were that low. **One in 10 born at the hospital endures withdrawal from some type of drug -- heroin, opiates, cocaine, alcohol or a combination of many."**

What are "Opioids"?

Given the nature of the subject, anything approaching a comprehensive answer to the question at the top of this page could alone be the basis of another book. And has by various other writers been so. However, such is not the aim of this book, and an in-depth understanding of the history, nature, and other aspects of opioids, is not necessary for grasping the truly serious status of our nation's opioid epidemic. No more so than an in-depth understanding of all things regarding automobiles, guns, etc., would be required to appreciate and guard against the dangers involved in their use and abuse. Hence, the following purposely briefed and relatively general explanation of **"what opioids are."**

Grossly over-simplified, **"opioids"** include a family of highly addictive **psychoactive drugs** used in treatment of mild to moderate to severe pain. Commonly prescribed in conjunction with surgery and dental procedures, etc. As well as often illegally used to experience unnatural pleasurable effects, feelings of euphoria, and other attempts to escape reality.

Opioids work by blocking or reducing the intensity of our body's natural transmission of pain signals to our brain. As **psychoactive drugs**, opioids therefore interfere with our natural brain function by altering our perception of reality, our mood, our thoughts, our judgement, our state of consciousness. Hence, they do not eliminate pain, they mask it. And any associated feelings of euphoria are — in reality — a most "temporary" and truly "imaginary" state of mind. **_Important to note_**: *Tobacco, alcohol, and cannabis (marijuana), are some of the many other examples of "psychoactive drugs".*

"Opioids" vs "Opiates"

The term **"opioids"** is increasingly used to refer to a wide range of drugs with opium-like or morphine-like effects. Whereas, traditionally, **"opiates"** can refer primarily to narcotic drugs naturally derived from **opium** (which is in turn derived from the seedpod of the opium poppy plant).

There are various classes of opioids. Three classes commonly referred to as narcotic or painkilling opioid drugs are: **natural** opiates; **semi-synthetic** opioids; and **synthetic** opioids. Listed below are some examples:

Natural opiates:
(Naturally occurring in opium resin of opium poppy plant.)
Codeine *(Used in making hydrocodone, etc.)*
Morphine *(Used in making hydromorphone, etc.)*
Thebaine *(Used in making oxymorphone, oxycodone, etc.)*

Semi-synthetic opioids:
(Derived from naturally occurring opiates and opium alkaloids, especially morphine and thebaine.)
Hydrocodone *(Brands: Lorcet, Lortab, Vicodin, Hycodan, etc.)*
Oxycodone *(Brands: OxyContin, Percocet, Oxecta, Roxicet, etc.)*
Heroin (diacetylmorphine) – *Declared illegal in U.S. in 1924.*
Hydromorphone *(Brands: Dilaudid, Exalgo, etc.)*
Oxymorphene *(Brands: Opana, etc.)*
Buprenorphine *(Brands: Suboxone, Zubsolv, Bunavail, etc.)*

Synthetic opioids:
(Fully-synthetic opioids synthesized from chemicals not derived from alkaloids found in opium.)
Meperidine *(Brands: Demerol, etc.)*
Fentanyl *(Brands: Duragesic, Sublimaze, Actiq, Fentora, etc.)*
Methadone *(Brands: Methadose, Dolophine, Diskets, etc.)*
Buprenorphine *(Brands: Subutex, Butrans, Buprenex, etc.)*

Among the other classes of opioids are those produced naturally in the human body. Such as **endorphins** secreted within our central nervous system to "naturally" regulate pain sensations throughout our body.

Why are opioids so often misused and abused? Primary among the many and varied reasons for their widespread misuse and abuse, is that, in addition to pain relief, at low to moderate doses opioids produce [temporary] feelings of euphoria. An unnatural "High" of intense joy and comfort, often without the intoxication, impairment, and other negative feelings generally associated with "Highs" from alcohol, marijuana, or hallucinogens, etc.

Risks from use: Opioids are generally safe if prescribed by a competent doctor and taken as prescribed for a brief time. However, even as prescribed by a doctor, regular use can for some result in dependence. Higher doses, misuse, and abuse, can also lead to addiction and/or fatality — where breathing is slowed, eventually to the point of death. Opioids are **especially dangerous** when taken with other central nervous system depressants, such as Xanax (alprazolam), which also slow breathing.

As earlier mentioned, as **psychoactive drugs**, opioids are among the chemical substances that primarily act upon the central nervous system. Where, as all **addictive-drugs** do in some manner, they alter brain function. Resulting in temporary changes in **perception, mood, consciousness, and behavior**. And as with all **addictive-drugs**, opioid-abuse can ultimately contribute to spiritual-bankruptcy; marital and parenting problems; difficulties in other personal relationships; problems at work; legal issues; finance problems; critical health issues; etc. And in sparing no aspect of human life, ultimately putting in jeopardy not only the life and otherwise well-being of the drug-abuser, but also that of their loved ones and affected others.

Drug "Schedules"

"Knowledge will forever govern ignorance, and a people who mean to be their own Governors, must arm themselves with the power knowledge gives." — James Madison (1751–1836), 4th U.S. President; hailed as "Father of the Constitution" for his key role in drafting the U.S. Constitution & the Bill of Rights.

Source: U.S. Drug Enforcement Administration (DEA)
https://www.dea.gov

The **Controlled Substances Act (CSA)** was signed into law by President Richard Nixon, as Title II of the Comprehensive Drug Abuse Prevention and Control Act of 1970. Establishing federal U.S. drug policy under which the manufacture, importation, possession, use and distribution of certain substances is regulated.

The CSA legislation created five Schedules (classifications), into which controlled substances are placed. Federal agencies such as the Drug Enforcement Administration, Department of Health and Human Services, and Food and Drug Administration, typically determine which substances are added to or removed from the various schedules, although the statute passed by Congress created the initial listing.

In determining into which schedule a drug or other substance should be placed, or whether a substance should be decontrolled or rescheduled, certain factors are required to be considered. Such as:

- Its actual or relative potential for abuse.
- Scientific evidence of its pharmacological effect, if known.
- The state of current scientific knowledge regarding the drug or other substance.
- Its history and current pattern of abuse.
- The scope, duration, and significance of abuse.
- What, if any, risk there is to the public health.
- Its psychic or physiological dependence liability.
- Whether the substance is an immediate precursor of a substance already CSA control.

The "abuse rate" is a determinate factor in the scheduling of the drug. For example, **Schedule I** drugs have a high potential for abuse and the potential to create severe psychological and/or physical dependence. As the drug schedule changes-- **Schedule II, Schedule III**, etc.—so does the abuse potential. **Schedule V** drugs represents the least potential for abuse.

The following is a brief description of Schedules I through V and some "examples" of controlled substances assigned to each:

Schedule I:

Schedule I drugs, substances, or chemicals are defined as drugs with no currently accepted medical use and a high potential for abuse. Some examples of Schedule I drugs are: Heroin, lysergic acid diethylamide (LSD), marijuana (cannabis), 3,4-methylenedioxymethamphetamine (ecstasy), methaqualone, and peyote.

Schedule II:

Schedule II drugs, substances, or chemicals are defined as drugs with a high potential for abuse, with use potentially leading to severe psychological or physical dependence. These drugs are also considered dangerous. Some examples of Schedule II drugs are: Combination products with less than 15 milligrams of hydrocodone per dosage unit (Vicodin), cocaine, methamphetamine, methadone, hydromorphone (Dilaudid), meperidine (Demerol), oxycodone (OxyContin), fentanyl, Dexedrine, Adderall, and Ritalin.

Schedule III:

Schedule III drugs, substances, or chemicals are defined as drugs with a moderate to low potential for physical and psychological dependence. Schedule III drugs abuse potential is less than Schedule I and Schedule II drugs but more than Schedule IV. Some examples of Schedule III drugs are: Products containing less than 90 milligrams of codeine per dosage unit (Tylenol with codeine), ketamine, anabolic steroids, testosterone.

Schedule IV:

Schedule IV drugs, substances, or chemicals are defined as drugs with a low potential for abuse and low risk of dependence. Some examples of Schedule IV drugs are: Xanax, Soma, Darvon, Darvocet, Valium, Ativan, Talwin, Ambien, Tramadol.

Schedule V:

Schedule V drugs, substances, or chemicals are defined as drugs with lower potential for abuse than Schedule IV and consist of preparations containing limited quantities of certain narcotics. Schedule V drugs are generally used for antidiarrheal, antitussive, and analgesic purposes. Some examples of Schedule V drugs are: Cough preparations with less than 200 milligrams of codeine or per 100 milliliters (Robitussin AC), Lomotil, Motofen, Lyrica, Parepectolin.

= = =

Note that the "example" drugs in the above Schedules I through V descriptions are but a snapshot of the actual numbers. A complete "alphabetical listing" of all currently controlled substances is available at https://www.dea.gov. A listing that as of December 01, 2016 included **"14 pages"** — being but another example of the magnitude and complexity of America's drug control challenge!

Especially note that, in addition to Heroin; LSD; Ecstasy; etc., **"Marijuana (cannabis)"** is also included in Schedule I — as State after State continue to legalize its within-our-nation farming, marketing, and use?

The "War on Drugs"

"Man's inhumanity to man makes countless thousands morn!"
— Robert Burns (1759-1796)

Addictive-drugs and their positive and negative effects have likely been with humankind since the beginning. For example, the Sumerians' (of ancient Babylonia) use of opium is reportedly traceable to 5000 B.C. And the earliest historical record of the production of alcohol is reportedly traceable to an Egyptian brewery in 3500 B.C. While the use of tobacco was reportedly introduced into Europe in 1493 by Columbus and his crew returning from America.

Just as additive-drugs have been around for ages, so have the struggles to deal with their negative effects. For example, in the A.D. 1500 timeframe, according to J.D. Rolleston, a British medical historian, a medieval Russian cure for drunkenness involved: *"taking a piece of pork, putting it secretly in a Jew's bed for nine days, and then giving it to the drunkard in pulverized form, who will turn away from drunkenness as a Jew would from Pork."*

And in A.D. 1650 timeframe, the use of tobacco was reportedly prohibited in Bavaria, Saxony, and Zurich. A prohibition nevertheless ineffective even in the face of the Ottoman Empire's decree of the death penalty for smoking tobacco. Even with the horrors and persecution by way of beheading, hanging, quartering, or crushing hands and feet, the passion for smoking tobacco still persisted. As it does for countless millions world-wide yet to this day!

Fast-forwarding a bit—as also noted in the *Introduction*, the United States first outlawed "addictive-drugs" in the early 1900s. And over 100 years later, our nation is now struggling with an ever-growing, out-of-control, addictive-drugs "epidemic"! Even after some 46 years ago declaring war—a "war on drugs"!

Our nation's "war on drugs" can be generally defined as a series of actions by the U.S. and other participating countries, aimed at ending the import, manufacture, sale, and use of, illegal drugs. Every U.S. President since Eisenhower has created "new" measures for decreasing drug use in the United States. However, the term "War on Drugs" seems to have been first used by President Richard Nixon on June, 17, 1971, when he described illegal drugs as being "public enemy number one in the United States."

The "war on drugs" has thereafter been continued by every U.S. President, by way of their respective tailored-versions of drug policy. During which countless billions of dollars have been spent, to no avail, in a yet to this day futile effort to eliminate the supply and use of "illegal" drugs—as well as the abuse of, addiction to, and deaths from, those that are "legal."

U.S. "drug policy" has a long and complex history. Below is a very briefed summary-listing of "but a few" events taken from a still-developing history. One leading to what is now, truly an "addictive-drugs epidemic"!

- **1800's:** Opium became popular after the American Civil War; followed by Cocaine in the **1880's**; and health drinks and remedies popularly included Coca. Heroin was used in treatment of respiratory illness; doctors routinely used morphine as a pain-reliever; and cocaine was an ingredient in Coca-Cola.

- **1806:** German chemist Friedrich Wilheim Adam Serturner isolated morphine from opium. Morphine soon became a key medical treatment in the U.S. throughout the 19th century, used treat pain, anxiety, respiratory problems, consumption, and women's ailments.

- **1853:** The hypodermic needle was invented, after which morphine began to be used in minor surgical procedures to treat neuralgia and gave rise to the medicalization of opioids.

- **By End of 19th Century:** Use and abuse of opium and cocaine reached epidemic levels.

- **By Beginning of 20th Century:** It became more widely recognized that psychotropic drugs have strong potential for causing addiction

- **1906:** The Pure Food and Drug Act required medical physicians to accurately label their medicines; with drugs no longer being thought of as harmless remedies for our aches and pains.

- **1914:** The Harrison At is passed, establishing the first U.S. federal drug policy; restricting manufacture and sale of marijuana, cocaine, heroin, and morphine; and calling for harsh punishment of doctors and pharmacists who prescribed drugs to addicts on "maintenance" programs.

- **1916:** A few years after Bayer stopped mass production of heroin due to hazardous use and dependence, German scientists at University of Frankfurt first synthesized oxycodone with hope that it would retain the analgesic effects of morphine and heroin with less dependence.

- **1919:** The Supreme Court ruled against maintenance of addicts as a legitimate method of treatment.

- **1924:** Heroin sales stopped with passage of The Heroin Act in 1924, making importation, manufacture, and possession, of heroin illegal in the U.S. Resulting from growing rates of addiction, The Heroin Act made even its medical use illegal.

- **1930:** U.S. Treasury Department created the Federal Bureau of Narcotics, increasingly criminalizing drugs.

- **1915-1938:** Over 5,000 doctors convicted and fined or jailed for prescribing drugs to addicts on "maintenance" programs.

- **1938:** Despite passage of The Food, Drug and Cosmetic Act, many medicines derived from opioids and already being sold, such as codeine, morphine, and oxycodone, were still allowed to be used by physicians.

- **1951:** Passage of the Boggs Act greatly increased penalties for marijuana use.

- **1956:** Passage of the Narcotics Control Act established the most punitive and repressive anti-narcotics legislation ever adopted by Congress; a heavily punitive drug policy with strong focus on law enforcement.

- **1940's-1950's:** Government anti-drug propaganda became so myth-based, exaggerated, and otherwise far-fetched, that many people started to doubt and not believe the warnings about drugs.

- **1950s:** Oxycodone became widely available when approved by the Federal Drug Administration (FDA) in 1950 as Percodan (oxycodone and aspirin tablets).

- **1960's:** Birth to a rebellious movement popularizing drug use and abuse to skyrocketing levels; a counterculture resulting in marijuana becoming fashionable on college campuses, and "hippies" using LSD in a search to expand their minds; with countless personnel returning from Vietnam War with marijuana and heroin habits and addictions. A resurgence in illegal heroin smuggled into U.S. was attributed to U.S. involvement in Vietnam. And since early 1960s, abuse of prescription opioids containing oxycodone has been a continuing problem in U.S.

- **1966:** Passage of the Narcotics Addict Rehabilitation Act by the Johnson Administration, specifying "narcotic addiction" to be a mental illness and paving the way for federal expenditures (tax dollars) for drug abuse treatment. With illegal drug use still considered a crime.

- **1970:** The Controlled Substances Act was passed and began to consolidate all regulated prescription narcotic/opioid drugs under existing federal law.

- **1971:** President Richard Nixon: (a.) declared war on drugs, proclaiming drug abuse to be "America's public enemy number one," (b.) called for drug abuse to be fought on both the **supply** and **demand** fronts; reflecting both the "temperance view" and "disease view" of addiction, and (c.) initiated the first significant federal funding for drug-addiction treatment programs. In a June 1971 speech before Congress, President Nixon declared in part, *"As long as there is a demand, there will be those willing to* *take the risks of meeting the demand."* By way of this statement, he in effect publically proclaimed that all efforts of interdiction and eradication are essentially destined to fail.

- **1973:** By Executive Order, President Nixon created the Drug Enforcement Agency, declaring that, *"America has the largest number of heroin addicts of any nation in the world. Heroin addiction is the most difficult to control and most socially destructive form of addiction in America today."* Thereafter, "Operation Intercept" was initiated, pressuring Mexico to regulate is marijuana growers, as U.S. government spent hundreds of millions of dollars securing our borders. Trade between U.S. and Mexico came to virtual standstill; resulting in at the time curtailment of Mexican supply of marijuana to U.S. – a supply quickly replaced, however, by a new supply from Columbia. Hence, thereafter, every effort to intercept the flow of drugs into the U.S. has resulted in establishment of a new route, through land, sea, and air. Validating President Nixon's earlier (June 1971) warning that closing our borders to drug smugglers is not a solution as long as our "internal demand" exists.

- **1976:** In his April 27, 1976, Special Message to Congress on drug abuse, President Gerald Ford declared in part, *"Drug abuse is a national problem. Our national well-being is at stake. The Federal Government – the Congress, the Executive Branch, and the Judicial Branch – State and local governments, and the private sector, must work together in a new and far more aggressive attack against drugs."*

- **1977:** President Carter called for decriminalization of marijuana; declaring within a speech before Congress, *"Penalties against possession of the drug should not be more damaging than the drug itself."* Hence, the Carter Administration's drug policy primarily focused on the supply front, with majority of funding spent on interdiction and eradication programs.

- **1978-1984:** U.S. cocaine use increased from an estimated 19 to 25 tons to an estimated 71 to 137 tons. In just six years, the "demand" had increased about 700 percent. And, with marijuana widely viewed as a feeder-drug to cocaine, federal and state governments began backing away from marijuana decriminalization.

- **1981:** President Reagan somewhat mirrored President Nixon's admission that fighting the "supply side" of drug abuse is a futile proposition, expressing that, *"It's far more effective if you take the customers away than if you try to take the drugs away from those who want to be customers."* Hence, President Reagan's "zero tolerance" program focused on getting tough on the "demand side" of our nation's drug problems. With funding for eradication and interdiction programs increasing from an annual average of some $437 million during the Carter Administration to about $1.4 billion during President Reagan's first term.

- **1983:** Vicodin (hydrocodone and acetaminophen) introduced to U.S. in 1978 by German pharmaceutical company, Knoll, became a generic formulation in 1983.

- **1984:** Cocaine was reportedly used regularly by 4 to 5 million people in the U.S., compared to 500,000 Americans reportedly addicted to heroin. During same time period, physicians explored use of prescription narcotics/opioids to treat cases of pain not due to terminal illness.

- **1989:** President George H. W. Bush officially initiated his version of the "war on drugs" on September 5, 1989, during the first prime-time address of his presidency. During which he outlined a federal government strategy of eliminating drug use. Through an approximate $8 billion plan (over $2 billion more than the previous budget) of which about 70 percent was for law enforcement and about 30 percent for drug prevention, education, and treatment.

- **1995:** President Clinton primarily continued the prior Republican administration's supply-sided drug policy; including additional tax dollars for use in both the demand and supply fronts of his administration's drug policy; doubling spending for prevention and rehabilitation programs, and making even more substantial increases for law enforcement and eradication programs. Of the more than $13 billion included in the 1995 budget for drug policy, about $8 billion was spent on supply-sided drug efforts, while only about $5.5 billion was spent on prevention, rehabilitation, and education.

- **2004:** In his January 20, 2004 address to Congress, President George W. Bush declared in part, *"We must stand with our families to help them raise healthy, responsible children. And when it comes to helping children make right choices, there is work for all of us to do. One of the worst decisions our children can make is to gamble their lives and futures on drugs. Our government is helping parents confront this problem with aggressive education, treatment, and law enforcement. Drug use in high school has declined by 11 percent over the past two years."*

- **2010:** In 2010 President Obama signed the Fair Sentencing Act (FSA), legislation that reduced the sentencing disparity between crack cocaine offences and powder cocaine offences, a disparity widely viewed to be racist. The expansion of addiction treatment was among the key drug policy aims of the Obama administration; evidenced in part by inclusion in the Affordable Care Act (ACA) [Obama Care] a requirement that insurers cover substance-related illnesses and mental health issues. And that individuals leaving prison be ensured access to drug treatment care after completing their sentences.

- **2014:** The U.S. bureau of Justice Statistics reported that 50 percent of inmates in federal prisons were there for drug offences.

- **2016:** In July 2016 President Obama signed the Comprehensive Addiction and Recovery Act (CARA), which aims to strengthen drug prevention, treatment, and recovery efforts. Legislation that provides for increased provision of naloxone, a synthetic drug similar to morphine, used to block the effects of opioids, especially opioid-overdose. Naloxone is increasingly being included in emergency-overdose response kits distributed to heroin and other opioid drug users and emergency responders. The price of a package of two auto-injectors has reportedly increased from about $600 in 2014 to some $4,500 in 2016.

- **2017:** President Donald Trump became the 45th U.S. President on January 20, 2017, and has promised to tackle America's fast-growing widespread use of illegal drugs. Beginning with securing our nation's borders against the flow of illegal drugs; and purging the U.S. of drug traffickers and other elements of the drug cartels, etc. Through a drug policy yet to be officially declared as of this writing. A no doubt very aggressive drug policy that will nonetheless be heavily challenged by an "addictive-drugs epidemic" and those benefitting from such. An epidemic surviving a so far lost "war on drugs" waged for many years by many administrations. At untold cost in terms of tax dollars; lost lives, and other human suffering. An epidemic that has now reached into every segment of society! A curse from which no one is truly immune!

= = =

"There are two primary choices in life: to accept conditions as they exist, or accept responsibility for changing them." – Denis Waitley

"Blunt force didn't knock out the drug epidemic. 21 million Americans are addicted to drugs or alcohol. And half of all federal inmates are in for drug crimes. People drink and do drugs for a reason. Cause it makes them feel good — until it doesn't anymore. The hallmark of addiction is that it changes your brain that's responsible for judgment. Prescription drugs and heroin act in similar ways on the brain. And, unfortunately, heroin, because of its widespread availability is a lot cheaper. One of the drivers of heroin has been the misuse of pain medication. If we're gonna deal with heroin and heroin use in the United States, we really have to focus on reducing the magnitude of the prescription drug use issue."
— Michael Botticelli (1958-), a Recovering Alcoholic; and Director of the White House Office of National Drug Control Policy, from 2014 until end of President Obama's term.

"It's better to fight for something than live for nothing."
                                        — George S. Patton

"When we go before Him, God will ask, "Where are your wounds?" And we will say, "I have no wounds." And God will ask, "Was there nothing worth fighting for?" — Reverend Allan Boesak

"It does not require a majority to prevail, but rather an irate, tireless minority keen to set brush fires in people's minds."
— Samuel Adams (1722-1803), American statesman; political philosopher; one of Founding Fathers of the United States.

Drug-Abuse:
The "Cause" & "Solution"

"Let us not seek the Republican answer or the Democratic answer, but the right answer. Let us not seek to fix the blame for the past. Let us accept our own responsibility for the future."

— John F. Kennedy

In the U.S. there seems to be three prevailing views about the root-cause of drug abuse, dependency, and addiction. In general terms they are as follows.

(1.) <u>The drug user is at fault</u>: In what is commonly referred to as the Moralist or Colonial view, the drug user is considered sinful and morally defective; and the drug itself is not viewed as being the problem. A drug policy under this view considers drug use a crime and calls for punitive measures against users.

(2.) <u>The drugs, drug-smugglers, and drug-dealers, are at fault</u>: In what is commonly referred to as the Temperance view, the drug itself is considered to be an addictive substance and basic cause of addiction. Therefore, a drug policy under this view focuses on drug smugglers and drug dealers as the "root cause" of drug addiction. To date, U.S. drug policy has been in large measure based on this view.

(3.) **Neither the drug user or drug supplier are at fault**: In what is commonly referred to as the Disease concept, drug-addiction is considered to be a treatable disease. Hence, a drug policy under this view calls for a primary focus on drug treatment and rehabilitation.

Ever since President Nixon declared America's first war on drugs, U.S. "drug policy" has been a subject of continuous debate and change. Whether of the political-left or political-right, some favor a policy of drug-criminalization and supply-sided focus. While still others push for drug-legalization.

Nevertheless, to date the **prevailing views** still fall within the three described above, with few significant changes over the many years. And as a result, federal funding of drug policy going in large measure towards drug **interdictions** and **eradication** efforts.

After years of democrat "and" republican administrations; a mix of drug policies and political agendas; an array of well-intentioned and ill-intentioned efforts; and untold billions of tax-payer dollars spent, little has really changed to date. **Other than the "War on Drugs" has essentially failed!**

And, as these year-2017 words are being written, the United States continues its struggle with an ever-growing, wide-spreading, out-of-control, **"addictive-drugs epidemic"**! One wherein—according to "two of the three" long-standing prevailing views—the **"cause"** rests with the drugs, drug-smugglers, drug-dealers, and drug-users. With the **"solution"** likewise calling for an effective focus on punitive measures against drug-smugglers, drug-dealers, and drug-users. However, to date the many-tried policies with such focus have clearly not been successful.

Therefore, could it be that the "majority prevailing-views" about drug abuse, dependency, and addiction, are off-target? Could it be that, in our tunnel-vision search for "cause" and "solution," we perhaps are failing to acknowledge and address the role that our **"demand from within"** may play? Demand from within our nation—and from within ourselves. Demand for both legal and illegal "addictive-drugs."

Could it be that, with less craving (demand) for unnatural escapes from the less pleasant realities of life, there would be less market for substances that destroy the more pleasant realities of life?   And that there just may not be a chemical (another pill) or punitive (punishment) **"solution"** to what may truly be a **"spiritual-bankruptcy problem"**?

Could it be that the self-destructive aspects of ignorance, apathy, complacency, denial, greed, and counter-productive fear, are road-blocking our ability and willingness to grasp the utter complexity of our nation's addictive-drugs epidemic? Blocking our ability to recognize the true root cause?

And that in addition to long-standing focus on the drug, drug-trafficker, and drug-abuser, our "drug policies" are failing to address the **"financial incentives"** associated with drug use, abuse, dependency, addiction, poor health, and ultimately death. Each stage of which, while being an **"expense and/or tragedy"** to one side of society, also represents a source of **"jobs; income; profit; positions of power and influence"** or otherwise **"justification for existence,"** to another.

Financial incentives driven, enabled, or otherwise enjoyed by, for example: the pharmaceutical industry; Social Security Disability insurance compensation; corrupt politicians and lobbyists; healthcare institutions; doctors incentivized in various ways to "prescribe medications," while not being afforded appropriate "time and resources" to diagnose addictive-drugs related illnesses; and, yes, even our charitable institutions; penal institutions; and the mortuary services industry; etc.

And as our long-ago **"War on Drugs"** continues; and as we citizens and our government continue to argue over law **enforcement** versus **prevention education** solutions; and as increasing billions of dollars continue to be spent on futile but politically rewarding programs and arrests; and as politicians, scholars, jurists, police officers, and doctors, argue over **prohibition** versus **decriminalization**; and as religious institutions continue to argue over whether alcohol and drug abuse is a **sin** or a **sickness**, and over how the sin—if it is seen as a sin—relates to the sickness; and as AA's Twelve-Step recovery programs continue to be the fastest growing "religion" of the day, . . . so also continues the increasing spread of our nation's **"addictive-drugs epidemic"**!

And so it will, until we as individuals and as a nation "truly acknowledge" this "threat to our survival." And likewise acknowledge that our search for and implementation of "solutions" — of "defenses" — must not only consider the root causes **within** our borders, but also those **within** our hearts, minds, and souls!

For, could it be, in the final analysis, we are likely to ultimately find that this worst-ever epidemic in our nation's history, is in large measure a consequence of our "spiritual bankruptcy" in one fashion or another?

And in closing this Section, and while trying to ensure constructive attention to the truly "daunting complexity" of our nation's addictive-drugs epidemic, four other likely barriers to our "solution efforts" come to mind. Obstacles that seem best expressed through the following six quotations:

"Rarely do we find men who willingly engage in hard, solid thinking. There is an almost universal quest for easy answers and half-baked solutions. Nothing pains some people more than having to think." — Martin Luther King, Jr. (1929-1968)

"The human mind isn't a terribly logical or consistent place. Most people, given the choice to face a hideous or terrifying truth or to conveniently avoid it, choose the convenience and peace of normality. That doesn't make them strong or weak people, or good or bad people. It just makes them people." — Jim Butcher (1971-)

"No one loves the messenger who brings bad news."
                              — Sophocles (497/496 BC–407/405 BC)

"Few men have virtue to withstand the highest bidder."
                              — George Washington (1731-1799)

"Darkness cannot drive out darkness; only light can do that. Hate cannot drive out hate; only love can do that."
                              — Martin Luther King Jr. (1929-1968)

"If you don't know where you are going, you'll end up someplace else." — Lawrence Peter "Yogi" Berra (1925-2015)

Brainwashing

> *"Is there any point in public debate in a society where hardly anyone has been taught how to think, while millions have been taught what to think?" — Peter Hitchens*
>
> *"Beware: open-mindedness will often say, 'Everything is permissible except a sharp opinion." — Criss Jami*

Any serious search for **root causes** of and **solutions** to our nation's **"addictive-drugs epidemic"** must not disregard the threat posed by **"brainwashing"** — commonly defined as:

(1.) A method for systematically changing attitudes or altering beliefs, originated in totalitarian countries, especially through the use of torture, **drugs**, or psychological-stress techniques; and **(2.)** Any method of controlled systematic indoctrination, especially one based on repetition or confusion, such as: through tailored advertising commercials; biased news media; political propaganda; etc.

As our nation struggles to deal with the complexities and heavy challenges of a wide-spreading "addictive-drugs" epidemic, clear-headed thinking is in critical demand. Clear-headed thinking that is in touch with reality and responsibly attentive to world events. Clear-headed thinking that is being in large measure smothered and overwhelmed by politically-biased news media, and by educational institutions that have become unrelenting arms of the radical political-left. As our young men continue to be emasculated; and our boys and girls continue to be **brainwashed** with **fatalistic propaganda**, such as:

- Life is or should be — fair;
- Humankind is gender-neutral;
- We are what we declare ourselves to be. For example, if one day I, the male, senior citizen, Caucasian author of this book decide to declare that I am an age 4, female, Chinese child seeking kindergarten enrollment and ladies-room access, the rest of the world is obliged to accommodate me;
- Achievement awards are "out" and participation trophies are "in"; and we are all "equal" in every respect;
- Truth must be replaced with political-correctness;
- Offensive words like "man," "woman," "male," "female," "boys," "girls," etc., must be removed from our government documents and educational materials;
- Hard work, sacrifice, contribution, making a lawful profit in business, etc., are not desired, required, nor respected behaviors;
- If you are not rich, you are a victim and it is not your fault;
- Everyone is deserving and entitled to an endless source of free stuff to be paid for by someone else;

- It is moral, ethical, and otherwise OK to burden future generations with national debt that is destructive of liberty, freedom, and opportunity;
- Political agendas preaching that we are hopeless victims, and separating us into opposing groups by race, religion, gender, ethnic origin, economic status, etc., have our best interests in mind;
- The government is the answer to our every need and want;
- While requiring a photo-ID for opening a bank account, cashing a check, or admittance into a hospital, etc., is considered sensible and accepted—requiring such before being allowed to vote for those running and leading our government is unreasonable, offensive, and being racist;
- We should never offend anyone—most of all, our enemies;
- Gun-Free Zones are "safe places"—respected and honored by the mentally-ill, robbers, murderers, and terrorists;
- A self-declared "fantasy safe-space" will not only shield us from hearing other points of view . . . but will also be respected by and protect us from our enemies—especially those such as the evil of radical/militant Islam;
- Marijuana, alcohol, and "prescribed medications," are not addictive or life threatening;
- The solution to our nation's addictive-drugs epidemic is simply to "legalize everything";
- The U.S. addictive-drugs epidemic either "does not exist" or "isn't all that bad"!

As such fatalistic propaganda is being spewed throughout the land, and too many of us continue to bury our heads in social media and other distractions . . . countless of the less fortunate elsewhere are being driven from their homes and their homeland. While others are executed; beheaded; drowned or burned alive in gages; raped; mutilated; imprisoned; tortured; having their fingers and hands chopped off; are thrown off of tall buildings to their death for being gay; used as sex slaves; used as suicide bombers; and subjected to other unspeakable atrocities! As thousands upon thousands of women and young girls are subjected to the unspeakable cruelties of female genital mutilation.

While here in the U.S., our continuing "War on Drugs"—waged many years ago—has to date been lost! At the cost of billions upon billions of hard-earned taxpayer dollars; and ever-growing numbers of lost lives, destroyed families, and other human suffering. The devastating consequences of addictive-drugs abuse, dependency, and addiction, that no amount of political-correctness and other "brainwashing" can ever truly mask the "reality" thereof!

= = =

"Our lives begin to end the day we become silent about things that matter." — *Plato (424/423 BC–348/347 BC)*

"If I were to remain silent, I'd be guilty of complicity."
— *Albert Einstein (1879–1955)*

Survival

> *"Learning is not compulsory . . . neither is survival."*
> — *W. Edwards Deming*
>
> *"We are driven by five genetic needs: survival, love and belonging, power, freedom, and fun."* — *William Glasser*

While the "rules of survival" are not "rocket-science" in complexity, for many reasons "surviving" is often a most daunting challenge. And for countless of our world's less fortunate, not achievable.

The Basic Rules of Survival:

- Threats to survival must be readily recognized and acknowledged;
- Effective defenses against each threat must be available or otherwise developed;
- The defenses must be timely and effectively executed to eliminate each threat.

These rules are a universal reality! Indisputable facts-of-life! Whether the threat to survival is a deadly virus; a weather disaster; a home-intruder; a corrupt or otherwise irresponsible government; radical/militant Islam; Sharia Law; . . . or **"addictive-drugs"**!

The above real-world examples are not noted in unawareness or disregard of the many other **threats** to our liberty, freedom, and ultimately our survival, such as: unsecured borders; failure to protect and assimilate common U.S. language (English) and common U.S. culture; uncontrolled immigration; inadequately-vetted immigrants/refugees; terrorism; out-of-control national debt; racism; political correctness; war, out-of-control Federal Government Agencies; cyber-attacks; politically-biased news media; politically-biased educational institutions; nuclear disaster; tyranny; dictatorship; military industrial complex; bigotry; radical-liberalism; radical-conservatism; expanding/over-reaching/intrusive federal government; mindset of deserve & entitled vs opportunity & earned; . . . and ignorance, apathy, complacency, denial, greed, and counter-productive fear, in dealing with our nation's **"addictive-drugs Epidemic"** and other threats to survival.

World history is cluttered with failed and failing nations that have not grasped and responsibly dealt with the basic "rules of survival." Over the ages, and yet today, untold millions from war-torn and otherwise destroyed nations have sought and continue to seek safe refuge — the opportunity to survive.

The opportunity for life, liberty, and pursuit of happiness elsewhere—anywhere—by any means available to them.

While countless blessed with this envy-of-the-world land of unequalled liberty, freedom, and opportunity, struggle with what has truly become an every-growing "national threat"—an "addictive-drugs epidemic"! One that continues its devastating spread as the result of our failures as "individuals," as "families," and as "a nation," to grasp and responsibly deal with the "basic rules of survival." Further enabled by the also threatening attitudes of many, that we are somehow immune to the devastating outcomes of the failed paths taken and experienced by others.

= = =

"I am not arrogant enough to tell you what the future holds, but I am faithful enough to remind you who holds the future."
— *Steve Maraboli (1975-)*

"You can present the material, but you can't make me care."
— *Bill Watterson*

"Live as if you were to die tomorrow; learn as if you were to live forever." — *Mahatma Gandhi (1869-1948)*

"When you reach the end of your rope, tie a knot in it and hang on."
— *Franklin D. Roosevelt (1882-1945)*

"Only a life lived for others is a life worthwhile."
— *Albert Einstein*

"You can't cross the sea merely by standing and staring at the water." — Rabindranath Tagore (1861-1941)

"Life is 10 percent what happens to you and 90 percent how you react to it." — Charles R. Swindoll (1934-)

"Refusal to believe until proof is given is a rational position; denial of all outside of our own limited experience is absurd."

— Annie Besant

"Let us not pray to be sheltered from dangers but to be fearless when facing them." — Rabindranath Tagore (1861-1941)

"Courage is what it takes to stand up and speak; courage is also what it takes to sit down and listen."

— Winston Churchill (1874-1965)

"A man can fail many times, but he isn't a failure until he begins to blame somebody else." — John Burroughs

"Religion is belief in someone else's experience.   Spirituality is having your own experience." — Deepak Chopra (1947-)

That is the definition of faith — acceptance of that which we imagine to be true, that which we cannot prove."

— Daniel "Dan" Brown (1964-)

"Your fear is 100% dependent on you for its survival."

— Steve Maraboli (1975-)

A Personal Reflection

"Life is about choices. Some we regret, some we're proud of. Some will haunt us forever. The message: We are what we chose to be."
— Graham Brown

"Everybody, sooner or later, sits down to a banquet of consequences." — Robert Louis Stevenson

"What lies behind us and what lies before us are tiny matters compared to what lies within us." — Ralph Waldo Emerson

At this point the special clarification earlier stressed in the *Preface* is worth repeating. That being, as used throughout this book, the term "addictive-drugs" applies to "all" of the ever-growing arsenal of mood and behavior altering substances that are physically-addictive and/or psychologically-addictive. Whether commonly called "illegal drugs," "legal prescription meds," "alcohol," "beer," "whiskey," "tobacco," "nicotine," "marijuana," "weed," "narcotics," "sedatives," "pain-killers," "opiates," "opioids," "heroin," or otherwise. For, again, our bodies are not threatened by "words" on a container or packaging, etc., but rather by the "real-world effects" from what we choose to subject our bodies to and invade it with.

And, like untold millions of others past and present, the subject of addictive-drugs is not a hypothetical, impersonal, or otherwise detached matter for various of my family, friends, acquaintances—nor me personally.

My drugs of choice were nicotine and alcohol. Nicotine by way of smokeless tobacco. After relatively brief stints with cigarettes, pipes, and cigars. And in my apparently hell-bent effort to get hooked on nicotine, an eventual choice viewed by many as being among the "less appealing" habits on Earth, finally worked for me—smokeless tobacco! My first "can" had a price tag of 19 cents; my last one (so far), about $1.25.

My routine alcohol of choice was primarily beer. And at times bourbon whiskey, generally at parties and in more formal social gatherings. While over the years, without ever developing a "taste" for such, I had on occasion tried about everything then available, such as, wine, scotch whiskey, vodka, gin, tequila, rum, brandy, etc. By the time I reached my then physical and emotional bottom, Xanax had been added to the list.

At the time, at least in the beginning, my drugs of choice were, in my view, considered natural "life-supplements." "Oil-on-the-threads-of-life," so to speak. Why, almost everyone, then or at some time in their life, to some extent drank some form of alcohol and used tobacco products of some nature. Or, at least to me it seemed so. And in my "dinosaur generation," commercials even included so-called "doctors" in white coats pushing various tobacco products. While tobacco company executives were swearing under-oath before our U.S. Congress that their tobacco (nicotine) products were not addictive. To say nothing about advertising then and now pushing the social acceptance of alcohol and prescription drugs.

But regardless of how things "seemed to me," in reality, and in the view of more attentive others, nicotine and alcohol were then, as they are now, addictive substances that alter one's mood, behavior, and judgement. And, in my case and millions of others, through abuse such substances can turn out to be not our "friends" — but "crutches". Destroyers of dignity and threats to spiritual foundation.

In looking back, such substances were social crutches progressively used and abused from my teens and into my forties. And, whether the substance was tobacco or alcohol, the "effect" rather than "taste" is what really mattered. The mood and behavior altering "effects" of nicotine and alcohol.

And in further hindsight, the warning signs were there early-on. Warnings that addictive-drugs were not something I responsibly handled. Early and later-on warnings ignored and denied throughout years of use, abuse, and other wrong behaviors. And not departed from until after hitting a physical and emotional wall. Until after making a "personal choice" to do so. A life-saving choice enabled by an addictive-drugs treatment program; Alcoholics Anonymous; support of my loving family; and the tolerance and accommodation of my employer and various others. But most regrettably, however, a choice made, and harmful behaviors not departed from, until leaving my loved ones and myself with ever-lasting psychological scars and painful memories. Not removable by even the most sincere expressions or demonstrations of apology, regret, and remorse, or by forgiveness by others. Nor by any thereafter well-intentioned deeds.

While our blessing of life does come with the power of choice (free will), it does not come equipped with a "reverse gear." In the final analysis, what any of us have is "this moment" and our "hopes for the next."

My selection and use of tobacco and alcohol was certainly not the outcome of any complex research endeavor, but simply the result of such at-the-time factors as availability convenience, peer associations, life style, etc. My "choices." And of course an abundance of ignorance, stupidity, and irresponsibility. Had any of my particular at-the-time life circumstances been different, and had today's vast array of drugs been early-on readily available, it is likely my addictive-drugs of choice could well have been quite different. As in turn could have been the ultimate outcome for me and others.

Xanax came into my life by way of legal prescription from a competent and respected medical doctor. A good man just trying to be of professional aid to a patient though troubled times. No doubt from the doctor's perspective, I represented a reasonably sensible, gainfully employed patient; a married man with children; member of the community; homeowner;

someone with a relatively responsible and sometimes especially demanding job; just someone in need of a little "temporary assist" in dealing with some of life's realities. A good doctor, whose well intentions by way of a Xanax prescription would, like nicotine and alcohol, also be abused.

The personal conduct of users and abusers of addictive drugs can and does vary widely from individual to individual. However, that some of the wrongs of various others surpass that of mine offers no meaningful comfort to me or to those I have hurt. Nor does such diminish my personal responsibility for my behavior, my choices, and my failings. For, whether clouded or not by addictive-drugs, one's choices are one's choices — as is one's responsibility for the consequences.

For the past 30 years I have been blessed to have chosen, one-day-at-time, to live life without the use of tobacco (nicotine) products, alcohol, Xanax, etc. And, when dental care and other medical procedures justify prescribed pain-killers (addictive-drugs), their use, if at all, is deliberately sparing, temporary, and with otherwise utmost care and caution. Behavior having absolutely nothing to do with "will-power," "strength," or "pure-living" — but a matter of informed and experienced "choice." A wish to be more responsible. To not put myself and my loved ones through the suffering I once did. A choice fittingly regretted for not always being made; one I am now blessed with drug-free opportunity to make.

Being blessed with a loving family, available to me always was the opportunity and responsibility — the choice — to treat them deservingly as "number one" in my life. Above jobs, above others, above human weaknesses—above all else. And there exists no words capable of expressing how deeply I, and no doubt they, will forever wish I had always done so. As better expressed within the quotations at the beginning of this Section—life is about choices. Some we regret, some we are proud of. And some will forever haunt not us alone, but also those whose lives we touch.

To fault "the substance" for our misdeeds and failings is likely a natural craving. A search for refuge. A temptation rooted in enlightenment of the fact that mood and behavior altering substances destructively cloud one's capacity for clear-headed thinking and responsible judgment. However, when entertaining such thoughts, it is crucial for all to recall that "past, present, and future" use of mood and behavior altering substances—the choice to drink, smoke, pop-pills, shoot-up, etc.—involved, involves, and will involve, just that! One's "choice"! Another of life's many inescapable realities.

Most certainly, my life-circumstances and past abuse of addictive-drugs are not unique or relatively remarkable in any way. Nonetheless it is hoped that this personal reflection is found supportive of the primary aims of this book. Which are, to in some meaningful way help draw constructive attention to our nation's wide-spreading addictive-drugs epidemic. To help eliminate the ignorance, apathy, complacency, denial, greed, and counter-productive fears, that continue to enable this truly self-destructive threat **"from within."** To be of aid to informed and responsible **"choices"** in our daily lives.

Choices free of preventable harm to ourselves and others. Choices that help us experience the blessings of life, through a body and mind unencumbered by the devastating effects of addictive-drugs. Choices that help protect and preserve life, liberty, and pursuit of happiness, for ourselves, our loved ones, and others whose paths we cross along our often taken-for-granted journey on Earth. A precious life-journey and Earth shared by others.

= = =

"May your choices reflect your hopes not your fears."
— *Nelson Mandela*

"The cost of a thing is the amount of what I call life which is required to be exchanged for it, immediately or in the long run."
— *Henry David Thoreau (1817 - 1862), American Author*

"I can't change the direction of the wind, but I can adjust my sails to always reach my destination." — *Jimmy Dean*

"Fall seven times, stand up eight." — *Japanese proverb*

"If you accept the expectations of others, especially negative ones, then you never will change the outcome." — *Michael Jordan*

"When was the last time you woke up and wished you'd had just one more drink the night before? I have never regretted not drinking. Say this to yourself, and you'll get through anything."
— *Meredith Bell*

"If you can quit for a day, you can quit for a lifetime."
          — Benjamin Alire Saenz

"The quickest way to run out of time is to think you have enough of it."   *— Stewart Stafford*

"Anger, resentment and jealously doesn't change the heart of others — it only changes yours."   *— Shannon L. Alder*

"I learned that courage was not the absence of fear, but the triumph over it. The brave man is not he who does not feel afraid, but he who conquers that fear."   *— Nelson Mandela*

"I never blame myself when I'm not hitting. I just blame the bat and if it keeps up, I change bats. After all, if I know it isn't my fault that I'm not hitting, how can I get mad at myself?"   *— Yogi Berra*

"When you blame others, you give up the power to change."
          — Robert Anthony

"You can't get away from yourself by moving from one place to another."   *— Ernest Hemingway*

So, You & Yours are Immune to Drug-Abuse?

> *"In my case, I learned that although God loves us, he doesn't grant us immunity from the consequences of our choices."*
> — *Donna Rice (1958-)*

Since in fact we are each and all relatively "unique" human beings, for us to actually think of ourselves as such—at least occasionally—would seem to be rather "normal." However, some thoughts of "uniqueness" can at times be dangerously self-deceiving; in fact, a threat to our survival. Such as, that we are in somehow immune to various pitfalls in life suffered by countless others among us.

Of course such thinking is but one real-world example of how we can and do at times become "detached from reality." Realities such as the potentially devastating consequences of the abuse of "addictive-drugs." And anytime that we get to seriously entertaining thoughts like, *"Oh, well, but that is something that won't or can't happen to me or my family,"* . . . it's time to get back in touch with "reality."

By opening our eyes, ears, hearts, and minds, to what is happening in the real-world around us! Happenings such as the few examples randomly-listed below. And as we review the following it is well that we keep a couple of considerations in mind. One being that the following examples are but a very minor snap-shot of untold millions of the past and present. Another consideration being that the following examples are in large part of people having fame, fortune, positions of power and influence, and access to the best mental and physical health-care that such can buy! Seemingly "advantages" typically not available to the countless more common among us.

= = =

Michael Phelps, Olympic gold medalist swimmer: In 2009, lost his endorsement contract with Kellogg's after photo emerge of him smoking marijuana. And once revealed that he "didn't want to see another day" during his long battle with alcohol abuse.

Michael Jackson, Singer; Songwriter: Died in 2009 of acute propofol and benzodiazepine intoxication.

Noelle Bush, daughter of former Florida Governor, Jeb Bush: Noelle Bush's drug addiction became public while her father was serving as Florida's governor, when she was arrested and struggled through court-ordered treatment.

Marion Barry, Former Mayor of Washington D.C.: Arrested in 1990 for crack cocaine possession; involved in one of the biggest political drug scandals in U.S. history.

Prince, Singer; Songwriter: Died in 2016 from overdose of the drug fentanyl.

Derek Boogaard, NHL Enforcer: Became addicted to prescription pain medication. A mix of oxycodone and alcohol led to his death in May, 2011.

Mel LeBlanc, Former Arlington City Council Member and Deputy Mayor: Found high on K2 (synthetic marijuana) and caught with a bag containing crystal meth and a glass pipe in his home. Some two weeks after returning from a drug detox center for addiction to methamphetamine and marijuana.

Lindsay Lohan, Actress: Her loss of control of her life included cocaine and alcohol abuse, DUI arrests, jail time, and multiple trips to rehab.

Josh Hamilton, MLB Player: His career was delayed and derailed for eight years as he struggled with drugs and alcohol.

Freddy Trump, President Donald Trump's brother: Struggled with alcoholism and died in 1981 at the age of 43.

Bob Bechel, Former political Campaign Manager, and Co-host of "The Five" on Fox News: Entered a rehab program in

2015 for treatment of a prescription pain medication addiction he developed after undergoing back surgery. Mr. Bechel has long ago publically acknowledged being a recovering alcoholic and his support of Alcoholics Anonymous.

River Phoenix, Actor: Exposed as a heroin addict after his death in 1993.

Jennifer Capriati, Child Tennis Prodigy: As a teenager, was arrested for shoplifting and marijuana possession.

David Hasselhoff, Actor: Began struggling with alcohol abuse in the early 1970s.

Anna Nicole Smith, Actress: Found dead at age 39 in 2007 with a lethal dose of a drug concoction in her system.

Steve Howe, MLB Player: Became the league's first player to be banned for life due to drug use.

Dustin Grubbs, Former Mayor of Poulan, Georgia: Arrested, charged, and sentenced, for possession of a bag filled with pills, including oxycodone and oxycontin—two different mixtures of Vicodin.

Don Rogers, Cleveland Browns Safety: Died of cocaine poisoning less than a week before his wedding.

Drew Barrymore, Actress: Motivated to get back on track with her career after two trips to rehab.

Mike Crapo, Senior Senator from Idaho: Arrested in 2012 for DUI in Arlington, Virginia.

Samuel L. Jackson, Actor: Started drinking alcohol and smoking marijuana and using LSD at college in the late 60s, and has said that until he "got clean" in 1991 — after a crack-induced meltdown that involved his eight-year-old daughter finding him passed out in the kitchen among his dime bags and paraphernalia. He had never set foot on stage without some kind of substance in his body.

Heath Ledger, Actress: Died in 2008 of a toxic combination of six prescription drugs.

Michael J. Fox, Actor: Turned to alcohol as an escape after a diagnosis of Parkinson's disease in 1991.

Trey Radel, Florida Representative: Pleaded guilty to misdemeanor possession of cocaine, after arrested for buying cocaine from undercover police.

Mary-Kate Olsen, Actress: Led to rehab by anorexia and related cocaine addiction.

Brian Wilson, Singer; Songwriter; Beach Boys front man: His drug-fueled descent into mental illness is the stuff of legend.

Farrah Fawcett, Actress: Suffered drug and alcohol addiction.

Macaulay Culkin, Actor: Arrested for Xanax and marijuana possession.

Elizabeth Taylor, Actress: Struggled with drug and alcohol dependency for years.

Kirsten Dunst, Actress: Has checked in and out of rehab for alcohol and drug abuse.

Rush Limbaugh, Conservative Radio-Commentator: In 2006 turned himself in to authorities on a warrant charging him with fraud to conceal information to obtain prescriptions; following a three-year investigation after he publicly acknowledged being addicted to pain medication and entered a rehabilitation program.

Elvis Presley, Singer; Actor: Died in 1977, reportedly from a heart attack. Toxicology results identified several pharmaceutical drugs in his system, with codeine being ten times the therapeutic level.

Carrie Fisher, Legendary Princess Leia Actress: Died in December 2016 from cardiac arrest, after recently relapsing from a long battle with drug and alcohol addiction, which include struggles with LSD and cocaine.

Robin Williams, Actor; Comedian: Died in 2014 while on antidepressant drugs. The antidepressant found in his toxicology test, Mirtazapine (Remeron), has 10 drug regulatory agency warnings citing suicidal ideation. His death ending more than 30 years of struggle with cocaine and alcohol addiction.

Michael Botticelli, a recovering alcoholic, and Director of the White House Office of National Drug Control Policy from 2014 until end of President Obama's term: Began drinking alcohol regularly in junior year of high school. By his 20s, was an alcoholic. Also experimented with cocaine and marijuana. Was arrested in 1988 for DUI following a traffic collision on a turnpike; a judge gave him the option of going into treatment or being sentenced to prison; he chose to enter treatment.

≈   ≈   ≈

As the above examples were read and pondered, and our respective life-circumstances were mentally compared, many if not most seriously questioned the soundness and sanity of any thoughts that any of us, or our loved ones, are in some way truly "immune" to similar fates. That is, other than those among us suffering from **"terminal-uniqueness."**

Otherwise, the above examples served a memory-jog that our blessing of free-will (choice) comes not with a blanket-exemption from the potential pitfalls of **"addictive-drugs."** And, when we are again tempted to entertain thoughts like, *"Oh, well, but circumstances and consequences like those above don't concern me or my family;" "We are above such behaviors and pitfalls;" "etc."* . . . then it is time and crucial that we depart from such threatening self-deception, and readily get back in touch with **"reality"**! It is truly hoped that something within this book is helpful towards that end, and if not, it is life-essential that we seek such enlightenment elsewhere.

= = =

*"The human spirit is more powerful than any drug and **THAT** is what needs to be nourished: with work, play, friendship, family. These are the things that matter."* – Robin Williams (1951-2014)

"I understood, through rehab, things about creating characters. I understood that creating whole people means knowing where we come from, how we can make a mistake and how we overcome things to make ourselves stronger."
– Samuel L. Jackson (1948-), Actor; Film Producer

"Substance abuse is a disease which doesn't go away overnight. I'm working hard to overcome it. I did fail my recent drug test. I'm prepared to face the consequences."
– Lindsay Lohan (1986-), Actress; Singer

"Sometimes you can only find Heaven by slowly backing away from Hell." *– Carrie Fisher (1956-2016), Actress; Writer; Humorist*

"When I was on drugs, there was a monstrous side to me, but I'm not really like that."
– Elton John (1947-), Musician; Singer-Songwriter; Composer.

"There's not a drug on Earth that can make life meaningful."
– Sarah Kane (1971-1999), English Playwright

"I'm one of 23 million Americans in recovery who have gone on to live productive Lives." *– Michael Botticelli*

The Guy in the Glass

by Dale Wimbrow, 1934

When you get what you want in your struggle for pelf,
And the world makes you King for a day,
Then go to the mirror and look at yourself,
And see what that guy has to say.

For it isn't your Father, or Mother, or Wife,
Who judgement upon you must pass.
The feller whose verdict counts most in your life
Is the guy staring back from the glass.

He's the feller to please, never mind all the rest,
For he's with you clear up to the end,
And you've passed your most dangerous, difficult test
If the guy in the glass is your friend.

You may be like Jack Horner and "chisel" a plum,
And think you're a wonderful guy,
But the man in the glass says you're only a bum
If you can't look him straight in the eye.

You can fool the whole world down the pathway of years,
And get pats on the back as you pass,
But your final reward will be heartaches and tears
If you've cheated the guy in the glass.

= = =

In grateful memory of the author, Dale Wimbrow (1895-1954)

= = =

Definition of "pelf": money; riches.

"Peace comes from within. Do not seek it without."

— Gautama Buddha

"Never ruin an apology with an excuse." –Benjamin Franklin

"If you can't forgive and forget, pick one." –Robert Brault

"Many of us crucify ourselves between two thieves — regret for the past and fear of the future." — Fulton Oursler

"One of the greatest regrets in life is being what others would want you to be, rather than being yourself." –Shannon L. Alder

"In this life, when you deny someone an apology, you will remember it at time you beg for forgiveness." — Toba Beta

"Right actions in the future are the best apologies for bad actions in the past." — Tryon Edwards

"To forgive is to set a prisoner free and discover that the prisoner was you." — Lewis B. Smedes

"We must all suffer from one of two pains: the pain of discipline or the pain of regret. The difference is discipline weighs ounces while regret weighs tons." –Jim Rohn

"Forgive yourself for your faults and your mistakes and move on."

— Les Brown

"When you forgive, you free your soul. But when you say I'm sorry, you free two souls." –Donald L. Hicks

Happiness

"This universe is balanced. God made it that way. There is always plenty to be worried and sad about, but there is equally plenty to be happy and at peace with. The choice is yours." — Steve Maraboli

"You live longer once you realize that any time spent being unhappy is wasted." — Ruth E. Renkl

"Happiness is when what you think, what you say, and what you do are in harmony." — Mahatma Gandhi (1869-1948)

It seems that regardless of good or poor health, wealth or poverty, good luck or misfortune, or the disparity of many other life-circumstances, some of us will forever consider our "glass to be half-full." While others among us will choose to see theirs as being "half-empty." Many take note of the overwhelming examples and other evidence that **"money"** and **"stuff"** may only for a while buy entertainment, comfort, convenience, attention, etc. While others seem convinced that such things are a lasting source of happiness or otherwise desired personal fulfillment. While millions of others seek happiness and other life-fulfillment through addictive-drugs.

And after all is said and done — or done and said — it is likely that Abraham Lincoln long ago touched upon a universal fact-of-life when he reportedly expressed . . . ***"Most folks are about as happy as they make up their minds to be."***

Nevertheless, the reality and wisdom of President Abraham Lincoln's above words come with at least a couple of often difficult challenges: "making up our minds" and "making the right choice." But thanks to our Creator, we have been blessed with the tool to do so . . . it's called, **"free-will."**

During some casual, good-natured small-talk with a lady I once had the many-years-ago opportunity to work with, I challenged her to come up with the **"recipe for happiness."** Within but a few minutes of me doing so, she handed me her hand-written response, which read: *"The recipe for Happiness: (1.) Something to do; (2.) Someone to love; (3.) Something to hope for.* Inserted below is a scanned-copy of the original:

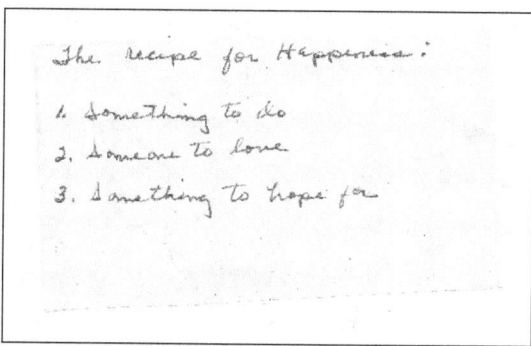

In an effort to put this little note into some proper perspective — it was written by a lady whose life-challenges at the time included, but by no means were limited to — the deaths of her husband, and thereafter a most special soul mate; considerable workplace pressures; special child-rearing concerns; and a life-threatening battle with breast cancer. Throughout which she never seemed to lose her faith, hope, sense of humor, work ethic, or "choice" to pursue her "recipe for happiness."

May something within this book be of meaningful support to your gift-of-life journey and pursuit of happiness!

= = =

"Do the best you can, and don't take life too serious." – Will Rogers

"If opportunity doesn't knock, build a door." – Milton Berle

"Failure is simply the opportunity to begin again, this time more intelligently." – Henry Ford

"The worst thing that happens to you may be the best thing for you if you don't let it get the best of you." – Will Rogers

"A pessimist sees the difficulty in every opportunity; and optimist sees the opportunity in every difficulty." – Winston Churchill

"There is a strange reluctance on the part of most people to admit they enjoy life." – William Lyon Phelps

"Most folks are about as happy as they make up their minds to be."
                                                    – Abraham Lincoln

"To understand is to forgive, even oneself." — *Alexander Chase*

"There is good and there is bad in every human heart, and it is the struggle of life to conquer the bad with the good." — *Susan Glaspell*

"The happiest people in the world are those who have the most interesting thoughts." — *William Lyon Phelps*

"Life isn't about waiting for the storm to pass, it's about learning to dance in the rain." — *Vivian Greene*

"Your fear is 100% dependent on you for its survival."
— *Steve Maraboli*

"Humor can be one of our best survival tools." — *Allen Klein*

"We need 4 hugs a day for survival. We need 8 hugs a day for maintenance. We need 12 hugs a day for growth." — *Virginia Satir*

"Take time to play! Ask for what you want. Laugh. Live loudly. Be avid. Learn a new thing. Be Yourself!" — *Mary Ann Radmacher*

"Be yourself; everyone else is already taken." — *Oscar Wilde*

"To make mistakes is human; to stumble is commonplace; to be able to laugh at yourself is maturity." — *William Arthur Ward*

"No one can make you feel inferior without your consent."
— *Eleanor Roosevelt*

"If you tell the truth, you don't have to remember anything."
— *Mark Twain*

"Your perspective on life comes from the cage you were held captive in." — *Shannon L. Alder*

"When dealing with critics always remember this: Critics judge things based on what is outside of their content of understanding."
— *Shannon L. Alder*

"We find comfort among those who agree with us — growth among those who don't." — *Frank Clark*

"You can never make someone like something they don't like, but you can always help them to better understand it." — *Criss Jami*

"Learn from yesterday, live for today, hope for tomorrow. The important thing is not to stop questioning." — *Albert Einstein*

"You've got to take the good with the bad, smile with the sad, love what you've got, and remember what you had. Always forgive, but never forget. Learn from mistakes, but never regret." – *Unknown*

"Attitude is a little thing that makes a big difference."
— *Winston Churchill*

"Not everything that counts can be counted, and not everything that can be counted counts." — *Albert Einstein*

"The only disability in life is a bad attitude." — *Scott Hamilton*

"Happiness can only be found if you can free yourself of all other distractions." — Saul Bellow

"Change the way you look at things and the things you look at change." — Wayne W. Dyer

"The best day of your life is the one on which you decide your life is your own. No apologies or excuses. No one to lean on, rely on, or blame. The gift is yours — it is an amazing journey — and you alone are responsible for the quality of it. This is the day your life really begins." — Bob Moawad

"I have not failed. I've just found 10,000 ways that won't work."
— Thomas A. Edison

"There are two primary choices in life: to accept conditions as they exist, or accept responsibility for changing them." — Denis Waitley

"If your ship doesn't come in, swim out to meet it!"
— Jonathan Winters

"You only live once, but if you do it right, once is enough."
— Mae West

"Being happy doesn't mean that everything is perfect. It means you've decided to look beyond the imperfections." — Gerard Way

"A sense of humor can help you overlook the unattractive, tolerate the unpleasant, cope with the unexpected, and smile through the unbearable." — Mose Waldoks

References & Suggested Reading

Book Titles	Authors
The Torah; Holy Bible; Qur'an (Koran) or other Religious Text of one's Faith or interest.	(Most literal translation and reader-friendly format of choice.)
The Faith Explained	Leo J. Trese
The Imitation Of Christ	Thomas A. Kempis
I'm Not OK. You're Not OK. But It's OK!	Chris Padgett
Alcoholics Anonymous: The Big Book	Bob Smith; Bill Wilson
Narcotics Anonymous	World Service Office
How *Al-Anon Works* for Families & Friends of Alcoholics	Al-Anon Family Groups
Codependent No More: How to Stop Controlling Others & Start Caring for Yourself	Melody Beattie
Words That Inspired Him — A Lifetime of Favorite Writings, Poems & Quotations	Norman Vincent Peal
All I Really Need To Know I Learned In Kindergarten	Robert Fulghum
Who Moved My Cheese?	Spencer Johnson
• Wisdom for a Woman • Wisdom for a Man	Gary Yarbrough, M.D.
• Mutterings Of An Old Man • I Felt The Floor Shake	Mike Womeldorff
Two Incomes and Still Broke?	Linda Kelley
• Threats To Our Liberty & Survival • Killing "Life, Liberty, & The Pursuit of Happiness"	William James Moore

References & Suggested Reading – *(Continued)*

Other References	Internet Websites
Alcoholics Anonymous	http://www.aa.org/
Narcotics Anonymous World Services	http://www.na.org/
AL-Anon Family Groups (Strength and hope for friends and families of problem drinkers)	http://al-anon.org/
Alateen — For Teens AL-Anon Family Groups	http://al-anon.alateen.org/for-alateen
National Institute on Drug Abuse for Teens	https://teens.drugabuse.gov/
D.A.R.E. Drug Abuse Assistance Education	http://www.dare.org/ starting-a-dare-program/
This Is America On Drugs: A Visual Guide	http://www.cnn.com/2016/09/23/ health/heroin-opioid-drug-overdose-deaths-visual-guide/
Foundation For A Drug-Free World	http://www.drugfreeworld.org/
National Institute On Alcohol Abuse and Alcoholism	https://www.niaaa.nih.gov/
National Institute On Drug Abuse	https://www.drugabuse.gov/ drugs-abuse/opioids
Drug Enforcement Administration	https://www.dea.gov/
National Drug Intelligence Center	https://www.justice.gov/archive/ndic/
Center for Disease Control and Prevention	https://www.cdc.gov/
U.S. Food & Drug Administration	http://www.fda.gov/Drugs/DrugSafety/ InformationbyDrugClass/

*"**Risk** more than others think is safe. **Care** more than others think is wise. **Dream** more than others think is practical. **Expect** more than others think is possible." –Claude Bissell (1916-2000)*

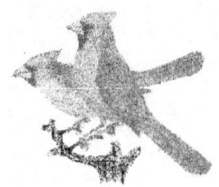

"It's not about time, it's about choices. How are you spending your choices?" –Beverly Adamo

"Never despair, but if you do, work on in despair."
Edmund Burke (1729 – 1797)

"Fear knocked at the door. Faith answered.
And lo, no one was there."
--Anonymous

"Enjoy the little things, for one day you may look back and realize they were the big things." — Robert Brault

♥

"As you admire the wonderful things God has made today, remember you're one of them, wonderful inside and out. You are blessed, you are special, you are loved." –Author Unknown

www.ingramcontent.com/pod-product-compliance
Lightning Source LLC
Chambersburg PA
CBHW062101280526
45788CB00003B/1309